The Secret to Manifesting Your Perfect Body: Weight Loss From the Inside Out

I0411710

Project Blissful

How I Lost 100 Pounds Without Starving, Sweating or Surgery

By Angela Atkinson

QueenBeeing.com

A BlissFire Media Production

Table of Contents

Dedication...4

Jump In: Project Blissful FAQ 5

What is Project Blissful?..5

What is a Bliss Mission? 5

What is a Fit Mission? 5

Who is behind Project Blissful?.............................5

Why did you create Project Blissful? 6

How did you lose 100 pounds? 6

Chapter One: Defining Your Personal Ideal State of Body Bliss
....7

Time to Talk About You...9

What It Feels Like to Lose 100 Pounds................9

How to succeed: Choose your own adventure.................15

Chapter Two: Get Your Sexy Back, Starting Today..............18

Get Your Sexy On, Right NOW..........................18

The Hard Truth: Like it or Not............................18

Chapter Three: Sneaky Skinny Secrets.............................20

Instantly De-Bloat and Appear 10 Pounds Thinner 20

Look Slimmer Instantly: Stand Up Straight..........................23

Look Slimmer Instantly: Change Your Hair 23

Look 10 Pounds Slimmer Instantly: It's All In Your Head
Anyway 24

Those Lovely Lady Lumps: Being Okay With Your Big Butt
....25

Look 10 Pounds Slimmer Instantly: Let's Talk About
Shapewear...27

Chapter 4: Drop the Weight, Not Your Life 28

How I Lost 100 Pounds and Still Loved My Life 28

My Very Best Weight Loss Tricks 29

Before and After Photos: Why You Need to Suck It Up and
Take Them...32

Fitness Mission: Take your own before & after weight loss
pictures 34

Affirm Your Weight Loss Success...................................35

Using Affirmations to Make the Healthy Food and Nutrition
Choices 36

Chapter 5: The Tracking Game 39

Food Tracking Tip #1: No Cheating (At First)...................39

Food Tracking Tip #2: Okay, Cheat a Little (Within Reason)
....39

Food Tracking Tip #3: Why Tracking Is Seriously Worth the Trouble...40

Food Tracking Tip #4: Find Your Inner Gamer (Dig Deep If You Gotta)...40

And Freedom From Food Tracking Looks Like This 41

How the Food Tracking-Game Changed My World 41

Chapter 6: Little-Known Secrets, Tried and True Tricks & Sneaky Shortcuts for Weight Loss....................................48

How to Lose Weight Fast Without Exercise Equipment.....52

The Dream Dress Method.................................57

Fitness Mission: Get Your Sexy (Fitness) On! 63

Chapter 7: Final Notes for Your Own Project Blissful 67

How to Stay Motivated When You Have a LOT to Lose 67

Sitting is the New Smoking 68

Discover This Surprising New Ingredient for Exercise Motivation..71

About the Author...78

Other Books By Angela Atkinson............................79

Connect With Life Coach Angela Atkinson........................81

Dedication

I dedicate this book to my daughter, Sophia, and to every little girl, teenager and adult woman who has felt "not good enough," whether it was because we were overweight, insecure, abused, broken or otherwise damaged. You need to know that it's not your fault, you can create swift and effective changes and it doesn't have to be painful. I have managed to learn to love myself healthier, and this book is my attempt to pay it forward and help you do the same.

Jump In: Project Blissful FAQ

What is Project Blissful?

Project Blissful is a movement toward whole-life healing, growth and improvement. It's more than a movement—it's a real whole-life project that anyone can join and participate in at anytime.

What is a Bliss Mission?

A Bliss Mission is an optional assignment that, if completed, could increase your own personal bliss by making your life just a little bit better. Learn more about Bliss Missions at QueenBeeing.com

What is a Fit Mission?

It's a Bliss Mission, but directly related to your physical fitness. Most of the time, your Fit Missions will just take a few moments of your time but with continued effort, can create real and lasting changes in your physical appearance.

Who is behind Project Blissful?

My name is Angela Atkinson, but you can call me Angie. I'm a certified life coach, a journalist, a blogger and the founder of

BlissFire Media, among other things. I also have three children, a husband, two cats, a home and a business to run. So I guess you can say I am just about like every other mom/wife/woman in the world these days - busy. And for me? It's all good.

Why did you create Project Blissful?

I'm a writer and editor (by trade and nature) who became a certified life coach in 2014, and have always found blogging to be somewhat therapeutic. I wrote this book because I know, without a doubt, that every single person alive has the potential and the ability to become the perfect versions of themselves. If I can in any way positively affect others in the world, it only comes back to me threefold. So, in addition to creating the Project to help others, I created it to help myself.

How did you lose 100 pounds?

It wasn't easy, I'm not going to lie. But I'm sharing all of my most important points in this book, and I am offering up my personal tips that have helped me to change my own lifestyle and drop the weight.

Chapter One: Defining Your Personal Ideal State of Body Bliss

"I personally battled with my own body image for years. I used to tell myself, You can't wear anything sleeveless or strapless. And all of a sudden I was like, What if I just didn't send such negative messages to my brain and said, wear it and enjoy it? And now I'm more comfortable in clothes than ever." ~Drew Barrymore

Do you struggle with your body image? If you do, you're far from alone. In fact, about 91 percent of women are unhappy with their bodies, according to a study published at DoSomething.org, a nonprofit that describes itself as "the country's largest not-for-profit for young people and social change."

Listen, I can relate. I have been there—and being human, I'm kinda still there sometimes. And according to researchers, only 5 percent of women naturally possess the body type often portrayed by Americans in the media. So what's a girl to do? How can you learn how to improve your body image?

I think you can and that's why I'm offering you a couple of free gifts (because I'm so grateful you decided to buy my book, and because it's stuff that'll help you meet your own weight loss goals. Pick up your free 5-day life-altering ecourse and ebook at this URL: http://queenbeeing.com/free-5-day-life-altering-course-attract-anything-want/

The fact is that how you feel about your body affects your confidence, overall self-concept and personal value. It is, whether we admit it out loud or not, a HUGE part of how we define ourselves, right?

It can be hard to feel okay about what you look like when you're constantly bombarded by insanely perfect images on TV, the internet, and magazines that depict people who are too thin or even (gasp!) digitally enhanced to mask flaws. It's just unrealistic!

But here's the deal. While we can't make that pressure go away, we can certainly decide how to respond to it. Stand up and recognize that you will be your most beautiful when you are your true self—not some random copy of the average Hollywood starlet/streetwalker/whateveritisthatmakesyouhateyourbody.

It's not just you—I know exactly how it feels. My body type has never been and never will be the Hollywood ideal. I am too short and my boobs are too small. Don't laugh! It's true. OH! And now, I'm too old (39). But I'm ok with it because I understand that no matter how much I worry and stress over the fact that I don't look awesome in most skinny jeans or that I have to buy a lot of my clothes in the juniors section (including sometimes bras!)–well, then I wouldn't have noticed all these awesome things about me.

Yeah, I know it sounds vain. But it's true–there are plenty of awesome things about me. But don't worry–I'm not going to list them. This whole thing isn't really about me–it's about you!

Time to Talk About You

So let's go there and talk about you. I'd lay money on the fact that there are probably lots of awesome things about YOU too.

So step outside of your head with me for a moment, won't you? Take a look at yourself from a whole new perspective. What are the beautiful things about you–inside and out?

What It Feels Like to Lose 100 Pounds

I used to weigh more than 100 pounds more than I do today. When you're as overweight as I used to be, people don't always look you in the eyes. They make assumptions about you that probably aren't true, including that you're lazy and unintelligent.

People who haven't struggled to get or stay slim don't

understand how it feels, but they are always congratulatory when they find out I've lost that much weight, which is nice.

Yeah, life's definitely different than it used to be.

People are nicer.

Like I said, overweight often equals overlooked. Since I've lost the weight, I notice that people people in general are nicer to me. They're more likely to offer me a hand or to smile at me in the aisle at the grocery store. I'm even more likely to get special discounts and other little goodies the world offers to petite blonde women. Imagine.

Truth? It makes me a little mad. But whatever.

Men are more aggressive.

Not that I'm complaining, mind you, but since I've lost the weight, not only do I get hit on more often, but the men (and a few women) have been a LOT more aggressive with their flirtation and attempts to gain my attention. This is mostly flattering but had been annoying/offensive and otherwise displeasing on a few occasions.

My feet are smaller.

I'd always been a size 7w in shoes, but after my second child was born, I found myself in a size 8w. I told myself it was related to the pregnancy, but interestingly, after I lost the weight, my feet quickly returned to their original size. (Score! An excuse to go shoe shopping!)

I can feel my bones.

Not like I'm super skinny, but for years, I didn't even know I had hip bones. Now, I can feel them. A weird thing to note (if you've never been overweight!)

I'm not perfect.

A lot of us think crazy stuff like, "if I could just lose 100 pounds, I'd be almost perfect! My weight is the bane of my existence!"

Truth? You're going to be just as messed up when you're done losing the weight—on the inside. So, in my case, I'm still evolving, and my guess is that I'm not alone. So I'm OK with not being perfect. Instead I work on being a perfect (read: best possible) version of myself in any given moment.

Sitting is better. So is standing. And everything else.

Not only can I pretzel myself into nearly any position, but I can sit comfortably almost anywhere—including on my husband's lap. And I can do just about anything I want with my body—I dig that. A lot.

I love my husband more, because I know he loves me for REAL.

See, when married me, I was 100 pounds heavier than I am now. And he still loved me and wanted to be with me.

No one else in the world can ever take his place, because I know for sure he loved me through some of the most unattractive years of my life. That is a beautiful trait to find in a man, no?

FASHION! Yep.

Listen, there are some really great designers out there who make out plus sized sisters look amazing. Unfortunately for me, being only 5' tall was working against me.

Some women can totally rock the plus size look, but for me? I wasn't pulling it off. So after losing the weight, my ability to wear and buy what I want has made life way more fun. And since I can now wear the day, s and m sizes depending on the outfit, I can get some really great deals on the clearance racks. (Around here, there are always leftovers in the little sizes).

I also shop the juniors section for some stuff. It's cheaper and for trendy items, works well with some pieces.

I still have to watch what I eat and pay attention to my body.

It's not a freaking cakewalk, people. IF you have been overweight, then you may once again go there if you're not careful. It's a matter of monitoring yourself closely and of CHANGING YOUR HABITS. That means it can't just be a "temp" fix—you've got to be in this thing for the long haul. So go ahead and have a little chocolate if you need it—but don't be crazy about it! Keep your serving size reasonable and make up the calories elsewhere.

Let's Start Here

I didn't share all the perks (and non-perks) of losing weight with you because I wanted to make you feel jealous or resentful. In fact, I shared it because I wanted you to FEEL it, even if for just a moment.

I want you to FEEL what it feels like to reach your ideal weight (or something close to it), because, if you can FEEL it, you can BE it. Stick with me, and I'll show you how.

You're not here to suffer.

The first thing you need to know about Project Blissful is that it's not just about losing weight. You aren't going to be starving, and you're not going to find yourself eating stuff you don't love.

They say losing weight is really hard. And if you want to look at it that way, I guess "they" are right–after all, you have to change your habits, your lifestyle and your mind if you're going to succeed. And exercise? It can suck. Plus, no one likes to be hungry, am I right?

But there's another way you can look at it. You don't have to fight to lose weight.

HOLD ON! Don't give up on me just yet. I'm making a valid point, I promise!

This is a very basic concept.

Why you can't lose weight: You are thinking about the fact that you "need to lose weight."

According to the law of attraction, whatever you think about and focus on is what you'll get more of in your life (to put it very simply).

So, if you are "fighting" to "get rid of the extra weight" or to "take off those last few pounds," guess what? You're attracting more of that to you.

More reasons to fight. More reasons to need to get rid of the extra weight. More taking off those last few pounds.

If you're telling yourself that you suck and you're beating the hell out of your psyche every time you work out–punishing yourself for letting yourself get out of shape in the first place—well, you'll attract more reasons to suck, more reasons to be mean to yourself, more being out of shape.

So, I guess what this means is that the Universe takes you quite literally—and negatives aren't a factor. SO, if you say something like, "I don't want to be fat," the Universe responds to "I want to be fat" instead.

See what I mean? Unfortunately, though, none of this actually equals to your being thinner or healthier, which is exactly my point.

You can't lose weight and keep it off if all you're thinking about is the fact that you are too heavy, flabby or whatever other negative qualities you're currently focusing on (and attracting to yourself in the process).

How to succeed: Choose your own adventure

It's as simple as "ask, believe, inspired action, receive." You have to first decide what you want the end result to be in your process. And be as specific as possible.

Try this exercise.

Ask: Choose your new body first. Imagine yourself at your goal weight. How does your body look? What can you do now that you couldn't do before? How does it feel when you interact with others? Do people treat you differently than before?

Believe: you have to first believe that you will meet your goal, and you have to already be there in your head. Imagine what it feels like to be in amazing shape when you meet your ultimate goal. What does it feel like when people notice you've lost weight and congratulate you? How do you feel? Why can't you start feeling it now? Just do it. Walk, talk and behave as though you have already made it to your goal. You will be surprised how quickly you can feel it if you try.

Inspired action: this is the part that some people get stuck on and that some law of attraction gurus fail to point out. But the fact of the matter is that you'll have to eat less and move more if you want to really get healthy, so when you're "there" in your head, ask yourself what your new, thinner, healthier self does. Do you dance? Do you workout at a gym or do Insanity in your living room? Or are you a runner, walker or biker? Does your thinner self Whatever your new, thinner self does to stay healthy—start doing that now.

Receive: meet your weight loss and fitness goals. Like I said before, once you "get there" in your head, your body will follow. You have to truly believe that it's working, and you can't expect it to suck (or it totally will). Instead, stay as positive as possible, keep your head away from negative, "fat" thoughts and become the person you want to be.

It really works if you work it. Are you ready?

Step One: Learn the Meaning of Unconditional

The truth is that a lot of us don't really understand what it means to give or even receive unconditional love. We assume our parents love us unconditionally when we're kids, but often, we're quickly disillusioned when we make the wrong choice one time too many. Same goes for our own kids, family members and friends - we think there's NOTHING that we (or they) could do to cause us to stop loving them, but deep down, we worry that there could be.

And then there's you, me - our Selves.

This is where it gets ugly.

We forget that we're worthy of love, let alone unconditional love. And if we look in the mirror, we might find it hard to fall in love with the person staring back at us.

Chapter Two: Get Your Sexy Back, Starting Today

Get Your Sexy On, Right NOW

Look, you don't need to start walking around in a bikini just yet, but if you're going to do this thing, then you must DO this thing. You must dress, behave and live as though you've already reached your goal weight. So what does that look like?

First and foremost, it looks a whole lot like confidence. And no, I am not going to start spouting the old standard self-help industry crap here - I'm going to give it to you straight.

The Hard Truth: Like it or Not

I learned the hard way that I could never really lose the weight and keep it off until I learned to be totally and completely okay with myself, flaws and all.

And once I got past the whole, "I hate everything about myself," crap that I muddled through as a teen, I realized this: I didn't hate myself at all. I mostly hated the fact that other people felt the need to judge me and/or try to tell me what I SHOULD be.

After that sunk in, I started noticing that I have some pretty cool qualities, and my guess is that you do too.

Mine were covered up by a few things - physically, obviously, my weight held me back in many ways, and psychologically, in so many more ways.

Learning to be "okay with who you are" can be much easier said than done, and we'll cover that in some detail in this book. But the most important thing to know is this: you have got to stop beating yourself up for your looks, your behavior and your life.

The only way you will ever be able to create positive change is to focus only on what you WANT, only on what you LOVE and only on what you're grateful for - even if you have to focus on the tiny, tiny things (or the big things - like the gift of life, for example, or of a home).

When you focus on the things that are good in your life, more good things are naturally attracted into your life.

So if you're focusing on having a hot, sexy body - even if that body is currently a bit plus-sized, you can totally have that hot, sexy body.

Chapter Three: Sneaky Skinny Secrets

Instantly De-Bloat and Appear 10 Pounds Thinner

I'm going to be honest with you—I've got issues with certain foods that I happen to enjoy. And since many of them are actually really healthy and good for me, I have to deal with occasional bloating.

When you're bloated, your entire body can seem to swell—and your tummy feels sort of like a puppy belly after chow time—tight and hard. It's also most likely a few inches fuller than usual and your jeans might start feeling a little painful around your midsection.

So here I was, sitting in a condo on the beach on the fourth day of vacation, feeling like I might be able to compete with the whales in the ocean. You see, thanks to a couple of changes in my routines, here I was, so bloated my usually comfortable jeans were cutting into my stomach—and the kids were begging me to join them and head out to the beach.

Needless to say, I was not looking forward to donning anything resembling a swimsuit with that vacay bloat poofing out my tummy and making me look and feel 10 pounds heavier!

So what could I do? How could I instantly relieve bloating and get my stomach back on track?

My jeans were feeling so tight they were cutting into my tummy. Admittedly, I had eaten a little differently than usual and I had consumed a few more alcoholic beverages–it was vacation, after all.

But I wanted to reduce that bloat RIGHT NOW in order to feel more comfortable, both physically and mentally (who wants a bloated tummy in a bikini?).

Here are the best tips I've learned over the years to quickly and even instantly relieve bloating in your stomach.

Try these DIY remedies to instantly relieve bloating in your tummy and abdominal area!

- Drink plenty of water–I know it might seem counter-intuitive, but when you feel bloated, drinking extra water can actually help reduce the bloat. You see, bloating is sometimes caused by dehydration. Your body thinks you won't give it the water it needs, so it holds on to the water it's got. Give it enough, and it'll release the salt and toxins that are causing you to bloat.
- Take simethicone capsules–Gas X, Phazyme, Mylicon or literally any store brand will work. This is the same stuff that they give to newborns who have gas, so you know it's fairly safe. I have had a ton of success with

reducing bloat pretty quickly with these low-cost OTC gel capsules. They usually work within an hour or so, but you might need to take another dose within a few hours. I have bought the store brand for as cheap as $3 for 20 capsules—and it works just as well as any other brand for me.

- Try a cleanse—I'm not going to advocate cleanses for everyone, because this can be dangerous for people with certain health concerns—so as with all other tips and advice in this book, you should always, always consult a medical professional before trying this at home. You can use almost any cleansing system, but I'll let you do your own research here. In the meantime, or to save some money, there's always the very effective and reasonably priced Walgreens Colon Cleanse. It's the generic form of a name brand, but it's half the price and it's totally worth it. Just be prepared to poop a lot!

- Doctor's advice for your body— Everyone's body is different, and depending on who you are and who you ask, there are hundreds of home remedies to instantly relieve bloating in your stomach. But whether you try one of Dr. Oz's many suggestions (among them, dandelion tea, water and magnesium) or you decide to go to your personal doctor to find the solution that is right for you, try asking your doctor or other healthcare practitioner if nothing else is working for you.

Look Slimmer Instantly: Stand Up Straight

We've all run across someone in our lives who told us to "stand up straight, young lady!" but not all of us paid attention or stuck with our good posture.

But I'm here to tell you—it matters. Here's why.

Healthcare and fitness professionals around the world are seeing scary trends that are directly associated with poor posture.

Not only do studies indicate that poor posture affects the way people perceive you, the way you perceive yourself and your physical health, but the longer-term effects of NOT standing up straight are downright shocking.

In fact, according to Eva DaSilva, a professional pilates and posture instructor, it's a real concern among those in the know.

"We're really afraid that this continual postural habit is going to create so many health issues in the future," she says.

Look Slimmer Instantly: Change Your Hair

Any good stylist will tell you that a change in your 'do can do wonders for your appearance and your attitude, but did you know that the right cut can actually make you appear much slimmer?

It's true! So go visit your stylist and tell her what you want!

Look 10 Pounds Slimmer Instantly: It's All In Your Head Anyway

Each of us is a product of her own thoughts. That is, when we spend time stressing about what we don't like and ignore those things we love about ourselves, we manifest more of those things we don't like.

For example, if we want to get thinner and healthier, we set out to lose weight. We think about losing weight, we talk about losing weight and we focus on losing weight. So, we lose weight…and we then talk about having lost it, and so on.

However, this kind of thinking can lead to temporary success at best–because when you're focusing on LOSING WEIGHT, you are bringing the need to lose weight back into your life, if you catch my drift.

Focusing on health instead, focusing on fitness, on feeling good…this is how to get there. Think in the affirmative–about what you WANT, not what you don't.

Those Lovely Lady Lumps: Being Okay With Your Big Butt

"I saw this beautiful girl the other day. She had an ass behind her that seemed to go on for days. In fact, I'm still going on about her." — Jarod Kintz, It Occurred to Me

Women, it's time to stop hating your bountiful derrieres and your curvy thighs. Big backsides are HOT, and there's never been a better time to have one.

As it turns out, not only do these two features make you more attractive to a majority of men, thanks to their biologically programmed preferences, but they may also indicate that you're smarter and in better health than your apple-shaped sisters.

Plus, scientists say, bottom-heavy women may also have extra protection against diabetes, heart disease and a host of other conditions associated with obesity.

Women with "larger than average" backsides were also found to be very resistant to chronic illnesses, University of Oxford researchers report.

Other key findings:

- Women with big butts have lower cholesterol levels and

are more likely to be able to metabolize sugar properly—that's why they're less likely to get diabetes.

- In order to maintain a "big" butt, your body requires an excess of Omega 3 fats, which catalyze brain development.
- Researchers found that children born to women with wide hips are statistically more intelligent than the children of slimmer-hipped women.

"I like big butts and I can not lie. You other brothers can't deny that when a girl walks in with an itty bitty waist and a round thing in your face, you get sprung." ~Sir Mix-a-Lot

Still, researchers say, some fat can still be very unhealthy. For example, belly fat can be a serious danger to your health.

And being extremely overweight, regardless of shape, is still fraught with health risks–so it's important to be healthy. But it's also incredibly important to LOVE YOUR BODY, the way it is, right now, in this moment.

And ladies…I'm going to be really, painfully honest with you here. As I may have mentioned like a hundred times, I have personally lost more than 100 pounds–and I still have a big, round butt. However, I don't hear any complaints about it. ☺

So love the skin you're in!

Look 10 Pounds Slimmer Instantly: Let's Talk About Shapewear

Despite tirades against Spanx by various bloggers in the fat-acceptance and the feminist niches, I am 100 percent for wearing shapewear–but only if YOU CHOOSE TO DO SO!

I personally will wear it all day long if it makes me feel better that day–and, a la Tyra Banks, I'll hike my skirt and show anyone who wants to see that right above my knees (or mid thigh, depending on the one I wear), I'm sporting Spanx (or whatever cheaper but equally effective brand I happen to buy). I won't however wear it if it makes me physically uncomfortable. I just can't–but that's why stuff like Spanx works so well–it doesn't "hurt" if you buy the right size.

So yep. There's that.

Chapter 4: Drop the Weight, Not Your Life

How I Lost 100 Pounds and Still Loved My Life

While there are plenty of folks who know how to lose 100 pounds, not all of them are writers or coaches, and not all of them are happy to share their secrets!

As part of my own Project Blissful, I've managed to take off 100 pounds (and counting!). I still have a few to go, and I'd like to invite you to join me on my journey. If you're not already there, go ahead and sign up for the free newsletter at http://queenbeeing.com to stay updated.

My name is Angela Atkinson, but you can call me Angie.

I'm a writer and editor (by trade and nature) and have always found blogging to be somewhat therapeutic—in fact, it's part of the way I managed to get where I am today.

And don't worry—I'm always thrilled to share the tips, tricks and general information that makes my own life easier. It's kind of a pay-it-forward thing.

Since I had my first child, I found myself struggling to keep my weight under control. After many, many fad diets (some that worked, some that didn't—none that produced lasting results) and gaining and losing the same few pounds over and over again, I finally GOT IT.

My Very Best Weight Loss Tricks

I've learned a few important things along the way, and I feel like it's my duty to share them. It took me a long time (and a LOT of failures) before I finally "got it," but if I can save even one woman from the wasted years I spent spinning my wheels, then this book will have served its purpose. If I can help even more? Even better. So, without further ado, here are my most basic tips - the ones on which I built my entire weight loss process.

1. Only Eat What You LOVE!

I am not capable of starving myself and I like food. So, one of my rules is to never eat anything I don't LOVE. (And, for the record, there are plenty of ways to do that without going crazy.)

2. Baby Steps!

I am not a fan of big, sweeping changes. So, I made one small change at a time to create more lasting results. It is TOTALLY working for me.

3. A Little Patience!

Lasting weight loss does not happen overnight. Like many diet gurus have said, it took more than a week to put the weight on, and it'll take more than a week to take it off.

4. Slow and Steady Wins the Race!

It's ok to go slowly when you're getting healthy. Even though I was losing weight more slowly than the people in some of my weight loss groups, the weight kept coming off. And even when I plateaued, I never gained more than a pound or two. Those who got into the fad diets and tried to be too restrictive are still at or near their starting weights, a year or more later.

5. Body & Soul Weight Loss = Fix Yourself From the Inside Out

My weight was a symptom of some things that I needed to deal with personally. I was literally "wearing my pain" on the outside. After a lot of soul-searching and internal work, the outside of me began to catch up with the inside—and I know that I'm not alone in those circumstances. That's why I created Project Blissful. I want to help other people discover and resolve their own issues and learn to be truly happy.

6. The Magic Pill

I hate to be the one to burst anyone's bubble—but there really is no "magic pill" or formula when it comes to losing weight. You have to eat less and move more—it's a fact. However, it doesn't have to suck. And, in fact, once you get going, it can make you feel pretty dang powerful.

7. What Not to Eat

I never eat mayonnaise, sour cream (unless it's reduced fat) or any other condiments that add fat/calories. I also skip the cheese most of the time. You would not believe the difference this small change makes.

8. Dress Skinny

Wearing "big shoes" as I call them (I prefer platform wedges, but anything will do) visually takes off ten pounds. Honest! But more specifically, you want to dress your body in the most flattering way possible. If you're apple-shaped, babydoll tops and skinny jeans are your friend. If you're pear or hourglass shaped, stay away from anything that isn't properly fitted to your body. If it's too tight, it'll give you the sausage look. Too loose? Think fridge-shaped person.

If you're not sure how to dress your body, send me a quick head-to-toe photo to angyatkinson@gmail.com and I'll send you some ideas for your body type. Or, just visit QueenBeeing.com for more style tips.

9. Self Confidence is Sexy. Be SEXY NOW.

I don't care if you have 10 pounds to lose or 150, you've got to love and accept yourself for how you are RIGHT NOW if you're ever going to get anywhere. So start here: every morning, from now on, wake up, clean yourself up and put on something presentable. I'm not talking about sweats and your husband's old t-shirt - wear something that you wouldn't mind wearing in public (the day you run into that guy from college who you still can't stop thinking about, maybe).

Do something with your hair, too, and don't forget a little moisturizer (at least) or, if you really want to wow yourself, do up your makeup, too. Sounds shallow, I know, but if you LOOK better you simply FEEL better. And people are nicer to you. Seriously, try it.

Before and After Photos: Why You Need to Suck It Up and Take Them

Do you take before and after fitness photos? If not, no pressure—but you should consider it, and let me explain why.

See, now that I've lost more than 100 pounds, I actually regret having deleted so many of my 'fat'/before photos over the years–I'm left with not so many to work with. But you can do better!

I don't know about you, but one of the things that has always inspired me when it comes to losing weight is "before and after" photos.

Whether they're mine or someone else's, I love to see them!

They literally prove that it can be done.

When I first started on my journey, I found myself googling things like "weight loss before and after photos" and "weight loss success stories."

I got on YouTube and watched videos that showed a progression of weight loss over time in photos. Those videos would later inspire me to make one of my own.

With that being said, there are very few full-body photos of me at my highest weight–and that's for a reason. Besides always hiding from the camera (or being the one behind it), I was a huge fan of deleting and/or cropping photos that I didn't like– and at that point, there weren't many I liked.

(It's true–you can look at my Facebook timeline photos I'm tagged in and probably guess when I was heavy–there are very few tagged of me from that time!)

Anyhoo, after I'd lost about 15 pounds, I did take some full body shots for posterity—one from the front, one from the side and one from the back. They are humiliating, and I wish I'd never looked that way—but I am so glad I have them now, because they offer me a reminder of how far I've come (and a reminder of why this is a lifestyle change and not a temporary deal.)

So, whether you're just starting your journey or you're already in maintenance mode, take some full-body shots of yourself—FOR yourself—today.

Fitness Mission: Take your own before & after weight loss pictures

Take three full-body photos of yourself today—one from the front, one from the side and one from the back. File them in a secret folder if you like—you never have to show them to anyone if you don't want to, they're just for you.

Weight Loss Progress Photo Tips:

- *Show as much skin as you can stand in the photo (but keep your private bits covered, in case you later decide to publish them or share them in a progress video like I did.) This is one regret I have—I wish I'd taken a couple shots in a swimsuit or at least something that showed more of my actual body.)*

- *Be sure you use a decent-quality camera if you can–but any camera will do if not.*
- *Try to take the photo in a well-lit area and remember that this is supposed to be a VERY HONEST photo–so let it all hang out. Not only will it give you a better idea of your progress later, but if you're like me, you'll find it very motivating.*

Do you find progress photos motivating in your weight-loss journey?

Affirm Your Weight Loss Success

When you have "convenience" food bombarding you from every direction, it can be difficult to choose options that give your body the nourishment it needs.

However, if you have daily reminders and effective tools at your disposal, you just may find that eating the right foods and feeding your body the best fuels becomes a lot easier.

Of course, there will always be temptation, but when you equip yourself with anti-temptation tools, you will be able to quickly re-focus your mind on your greater goal of getting healthy!

Using Affirmations to Make the Healthy Food and Nutrition Choices

When everyone around you at the office is indulging in burgers, fries, and sugary drinks, it's awfully tempting to join in, isn't it?

But what if you could stop that temptation in its tracks and actually choose to make a healthy choice? You don't need me to tell you that fatty and sugary choices are not the kinds of food that your body needs – you need to tell yourself!

It can be hard in moments of temptation to make the right choice, but with the help of positive affirmations, you can retrain your brain to replace the desire for junk food with healthy choices.

Affirmations can help you stick to your diet, say no to temptation, and eat nourishing and satisfying foods. How? By replacing the negative spiral of thoughts in your mind with powerful, positive ones.

But first you have to believe that it is possible to gain control over your thirsts, desires, and cravings. The first step in making a lasting change in your life is to make the commitment to success. Are you committed? Do you believe that you can overcome your cravings?

Once you've set your commitment in stone, you're ready to learn the top 10 affirmations to get you through moments of weakness.

Top 10 Food and Nutrition Affirmations

Before reading the list below, you should know that affirmations are most successful when you internalize the saying and repeat it frequently. Whether you're having a good or bad day, you need to be constantly repeating these positive statements in your mind. Temptation will strike when you least expect it, so it's better to be prepared!

1. I can neutralize bad habits with good food, exercise, and healthy living.
2. I am proud to reach out to my support network instead of leaning on food for comfort.
3. I am losing weight for me because I love me.
4. I set aside time just for me.
5. My good health and productivity are the rewards for the nourishing foods I eat.
6. Weight gain happens over time, so my weight loss equally requires time, patience, and lifestyle changes.
7. I use self-care, not self-control.
8. The more I take care of myself, the better I feel.
9. I am firmly committed to staying active and healthy.
10. I deserve a healthy body and mind.

When you look at these food and nutrition affirmations, they may seem like ideals – behaviors and thoughts that you only wish you could have – but each time you reaffirm them by saying them aloud, you're slowly changing your mindset. Over time, these ideals will become a reality through your thoughts and actions.

But remember, you must first believe you can change. Once you make the commitment to your success, you will change your attitudes about food and you'll be thankful you did!

Chapter 5: The Tracking Game

Tracking your food is a huge pain in the ass. I'm not gonna lie.

But if you can do it for a month, you can do it for six months.

And often times, if you do it for six months, you don't have to keep doing it all the time.

Food Tracking Tip #1: No Cheating (At First)

I had to be very strict about tracking during the beginning in order to lose the weight. I had to track every day for at least six months before I felt like I was ready to try going track free.

I tracked every single thing I put in my mouth—even if it was just a handful of peanuts or a bite of a cookie. It mattered, and it changed my life.

Food Tracking Tip #2: Okay, Cheat a Little (Within Reason)

Some people do well with a "cheat day" each week, others need two. My suggestion is to do one or less "days" of "freedom" at first.

Instead, I suggest a "cheat meal" option or a "cheat dessert" option once a week.

For me, the Weight Watchers bonus points (aka cheat within

reason option) made it easier to understand what an appropriate amount of cheating looked like, and tracking taught me how to eat right and still live in the "real world."

But even when you cheat, you should still track every single thing you eat. It will help to know exactly what kind of damage you're doing–in more ways than one.

Food Tracking Tip #3: Why Tracking Is Seriously Worth the Trouble

Look, I know what you're thinking. Tracking food? Boring, waste of time, annoying, restrictive, waste of energy–doesn't work anyway. Right?

Wrong. So wrong.

For me, tracking everything I ate and drank was a pain at first and felt really restrictive, but that short period of restriction ultimately led to freedom.

It will be for you too, I promise–so just do it!

Food Tracking Tip #4: Find Your Inner Gamer (Dig Deep If You Gotta)

So listen, I'm not a gamer. Honestly. But tracking sort of became a game to me, eventually. I actually (don't tell anyone) sort of had fun with it.

I wanted to see how much I could eat while still staying within my points allowance, so I'd figure out different menu options and play with the numbers until I had the most satisfying options possible. Give it a shot!

And Freedom From Food Tracking Looks Like This

These days, I don't track on a daily basis. But through tracking, I learned what portion sizes are healthier, which small adjustments to which dishes can reduce your fat and calories but still retain the flavor and more.

But the biggest and most important thing that six months of tracking my food helped me to learn was how to listen to my own body's cues.

Now, I just eat what I want and nothing more or less. I pay attention to my body and feed it what it wants—and nothing else.

How the Food Tracking-Game Changed My World

Within the confines of my little game, I naturally leaned toward healthier foods. Fruits and veggies were mostly free—so I could eat a HUGE and awesome salad with a few ounces of chicken and a couple tablespoons of dressing for seven or eight points, max.

This kind of game-playing led to a change in my taste preferences. Eating greasy, cheesy, creamy, fried or otherwise bad-for-me foods suddenly became less attractive.

Now, I wanted fresh, cleaner-tasting stuff.

These days, I am able to literally eat anything I want, simply by eating healthy MOST of the time and by allowing myself to indulge on occasion.

And since I'm still working on getting those last few pounds off, I am still keeping an eye on my scale. If I notice that I plateau for too long or even gain a pound or two, I'll go back to tracking for a few weeks so I can regain balance.

Fitness Mission: Make a game of it!

I promise, tracking your food doesn't have to (totally) suck. You might be surprised to find out how much (or how little) you're really eating and how small changes in your choices can lead to big changes in your health.

Supercharge Your Weight Loss

Truth be told, there's not really anything most would consider particularly easy about weight loss—but there are some things you can do to make it go a little more smoothly. And good news—there are several easy ways to boost your metabolism that you can try without much exercise.

Here are some really simple "life tweaks" you can use to speed up your metabolism.

"The higher your energy level, the more efficient your body. The more efficient your body, the better you feel and the more you will use your talent to produce outstanding results."
~Anthony Robbins

You know that your health is important, and that daily exercise can cut your risk of disease while dramatically increasing your energy. But how do you fit a workout into your busy schedule? Are you too tired after a hard day of work to take advantage of a gym membership? Thankfully, it's possible to stay fit without missing a beat of your busy lifestyle.

Who needs expensive, cumbersome exercise equipment or the daily commute to the gym, when you can get valuable, heart pumping exercise almost anywhere?

When to Give Yourself a Break: No Deprivation Allowed!

"Everything in moderation, including moderation."— Oscar *Wilde*

Listen, I've always said I don't like feeling deprived. I could never lose weight on a consistent basis until I figured out that doing it right didn't mean ALWAYS eating right. It meant eating right most of the time, and just paying attention to how much I ate all the time.

Bottom line, if you love food and you don't want to live on lettuce and carrots, it's all about HOW MUCH you eat, not necessarily WHAT. As long as it all adds up to a calorie deficit by the end of the day, you're all set for weight loss. If not, at least burn as much as you take in—and you won't gain any weight when you splurge a little.

Portion control is key to losing weight without feeling deprived.

You can eat chocolate cake and other foods you love if you just reduce the serving size. Try these strategies to reduce your portion sizes and lose those extra pounds.

Tips for Eating at Home

1. **Plan weekly menus.** Sketch out your eating plan for a week at a time and use it to guide your grocery shopping. Many people underestimate how much they eat. This system will make any discrepancies obvious. If you run out of food before the end of the week, you may need to re-evaluate your diet.
2. **Read the package labels.** It's easy to assume that convenience foods would be packaged in single servings. Check the label to be sure. A single bottle of

juice often contains 2 or more servings, so find out how many calories you're really consuming.

3. **Learn to eyeball.** A three-ounce portion of grilled fish is about the size of a deck of playing cards. A cup of breakfast cereal looks about as big as a tennis ball. You may want to measure and weigh your favorite foods while you're learning to visually estimate portions.

4. **Count your bites.** Counting each bite is another temporary method that can help. Notice how many bites you're eating. By eating more mindfully, you may find that your taste buds are satisfied with just a few spoonfuls of ice cream.

5. **Divvy up your plate.** As you learn to visually estimate portions, you'll discover about how much of your plate they typically cover. Keep this in mind when you dish up your food. Health experts recommend that most adults get about 2 to 3 cups of vegetables daily, so get used to giving them the most room.

6. **Use smaller dishes.** Smaller plates and bowls will make servings look more generous. Keep big platters off the table to remove the temptation to help yourself to more. When snacking, put just a few chips in your bowl at a time. Force yourself to walk back to the kitchen again if you want more.

7. **Package or freeze leftovers.** You can save time by baking big batches of lasagna. Just put the leftovers in

the freezer right away so that you don't succumb to the temptation to have just a little more.

Tips for Dining Out:

1. **Set aside leftovers immediately.** The same strategy works when you're eating out. Cut your hamburger in half and push the remainder to the side. If your powers of resistance need a little support, ask ahead for half of your meal to be packed to go.

2. **Ask for sauces on the side.** Sauces and dressings can add a lot of calories to otherwise healthy dishes. Request that condiments be served on the side so you can control how much you use.

3. **Order the smallest size.** You can minimize the damage at fast food places by ordering the smallest size on the menu. Hot French fries taste better so you can actually have a more satisfying experience by eating less.

4. **Share a meal with a friend.** Splitting a meal is often more fun than having leftovers. Ask your server to divide it or just bring two spoons if you're very close friends.

5. **Ask questions.** Some items are obviously dangerous to your diet, but others may require clarification. Ask what's in the salad or how big the seafood platter is. You may want to leave out the bacon or decide that the

appetizer has enough calories for a whole meal.

These new eating habits are effective and easy to learn. By reducing your portions sizes, you can manage your weight while enjoying a wide variety of delicious and healthy foods.

Chapter 6: Little-Known Secrets, Tried and True Tricks & Sneaky Shortcuts for Weight Loss

Let's Talk About My Abs: Here is Where I Reveal ALL of My Tummy Secrets!

As a mother of three children who spanned over 10 years (and who were each born by cesarean section) and a woman who has lost more than 100 pounds, you wouldn't expect that my mid-section would look very good.

But over the months, I've managed to shave off inches and have actually managed to develop fairly defined ab muscles. You can take a look at them at QueenBeeing.com/angies-abs, if you want to see what I'm talking about.

Anyway, a couple of months ago when I first felt nervy enough to post the pics on Facebook, my friends begged me to tell them my secrets. I promised that I would spill the beans in my upcoming book, so here we go.

Secret #1: Isometric Exercises

I hate situps. In fact, I don't really like any kind of exercise that makes me lay on the floor. (Yeah, I'm one of those "glamping" types of people - camping is way too dirty for me!)

Anyway, I digress. Over the years, I've learned that simply tightening and releasing the muscles in your stomach can be significant in creating the appearance of a flat stomach and abs.

Start by practicing in the car. Whenever you're at a stoplight, tighten and hold your abdominal muscles for 10 seconds, then release for 10. Do this until the light turns green. As it becomes more comfortable, you can add it to other areas of your life.

I find that tightening my stomach muscles while walking and carrying weights is incredibly effective, and doing so while performing arm exercises will help to define them more quickly.

Basically, the more you do it and the more often, the more quickly you'll see results. I tend to do it almost all the time now, and especially near cameras. (Only halfway joking!)

Secret #2: Coconut Oil in My Coffee

So I had read a bunch of studies about how coconut oil was beneficial for losing belly fat somehow, and after doing my research, I decided it couldn't hurt. I bought a jar of the stuff for $8 at Target and got started.

It's a little more than a hundred calories per serving, so I had to take that into consideration, but when I looked at all of the potential benefits, I couldn't pass up the opportunity to try it.

It definitely seemed to help to make my abs appear more defined and may have also offered some other benefits healthwise. One thing was clear: I felt a certain amount of "cleansing" action for a day or so after the initial doses.

The reason I tried it and recommend it to my clients today (though I am a coach, not a medical professional - so you should always check with your doctor before trying these or any other weight loss regimens) is because it worked for me, it cost me very little to try and it is a natural food product, not some chemical that has unknown side effects.

Another well-documented benefit of taking coconut oil: the lack of hunger factor. Somehow coconut oil reduces your appetite (at least when your body doesn't really need food). I experienced it myself, and that was why I continued to use the stuff - even though it added calories to my coffee, it removed them from my day overall.

You don't have to put it in your coffee, of course - though I think it tastes lovely that way. Some people blend it into a smoothie, others add it to tea or even to their oatmeal in the morning. You can even use it in place of other cooking oils.

It's worth a shot, and it helped me. My advice to you?

As long as you're not allergic to coconut and you have your doc's approval, this is a safe way to go. Just be careful to limit yourself to 3 to 5 tablespoons per day AND to take those calories into account.

Secret #3: Moisturize and Massage

Your stomach will look tighter and less bloated if you use good moisturizer on it and massage it firmly each day. Sounds like it isn't a big deal, but try it for a month and then get back to me. Even those women with the worst stretch marks can benefit from this simple and effective secret.

And like I mentioned before - using a product like Vick's Vapor Rub now and then will help firm it up too - but this is a primarily cosmetic tip. Even so, sticking to it can help reduce your midsection by inches.

Secret #4: Shapewear

Did you know that wearing shapewear like Spanx on the regular can actually help to reshape your body? It's true. Consider it a far less painful version of corseting, if you will. It works even better with secret #3 in play too.

Secret #5: Considering Consumption

Certain foods, drinks and behaviors are going to cause your tummy to bloat and look less flat. So if you can identify those and reduce or eliminate them from your life, you can have a bit more control over your level of bloat and avoid extra inches.

Bubbly drinks like soda, good-for-you veggies and legumes and even white flour are all food culprits for unnecessary bloating. Find out which ones are triggers for you and only eat them when you don't have to go out in the world.

Other things to consider - drinking through a straw, gulping your food, screaming a lot or even just being very dramatic (sighing a lot!) can cause you to take air into your stomach and can make you feel uncomfortable and bloaty.

How to Lose Weight Fast Without Exercise Equipment

Try these easy tips to get and stay fit around your home or workplace:

Take a walk. Walking is one of the most accessible forms of exercise. You can incorporate more steps into your day by simply walking around the block during lunchtime or taking the stairs instead of the elevator. Even if you exercise regularly at a gym, walking can supplement your routine for more energy and a leaner body.

Tip: Consider purchasing a pedometer that counts your steps. Wear it all day, and write down the number of steps you've taken at the end of the day. Each week, set a daily goal of steps and increase that goal each week. You'll be surprised how your mind finds ways to get more steps into your daily routine.

Try a body wrap and get your greens. Certain herb-and-plant-based nutritional supplements and products are aimed at helping to slim you down and tone you up without any exercise at all. While there are some that are primarily made up of diuretics and laxatives, there are plenty of all-natural options out there.

LITTLE KNOWN SECRET: Don't tell anyone I told you this, but applying a nice thick coat of Vick's Vapor Rub or a similar product will help shrink up loose skin just as well as most body wraps. Shh!

Practice breathing exercises. As often as possible, focus on your breathing. Learning to relax and slow down your breathing will do wonders for your physical and mental health. You'll handle stress better and meet the challenges of your life with more effective responses when you learn to relax under pressure by focusing on your breathing.

- *Tip: You can focus on your breathing anywhere. When you're stuck at a red light, use the time to relax, instead of getting frustrated at the delay. In between activities or duties at work, take a breathing break. And, when you start to feel stressed, take just a few seconds to breathe deeply and refocus on solutions. Use this technique: Close your eyes (if you're not driving, of course), and slowly inhale through your nose. Then exhale slowly through your mouth, pause, and repeat a few times. Place your hand on your stomach, covering your belly button. If you're breathing correctly, your hand will slowly rise and fall.*

Drink lots of water and eat nutritiously. Drink as much water as possible to keep your body well hydrated and functioning at peak efficiency. Think of the food you put into your body as fuel for your life, and choose to fuel your body with high-energy foods that keep you fit.

- *Tip: Eat as many fresh fruits and vegetables as possible. Fill your dinner plate with vegetables and a smaller portion of meat and carbohydrates. Eat fruits for an energy-producing alternative to candy bars or other sugary snacks.*

Exercise for at least 10 minutes per day. You can exercise anywhere, without using special equipment. Examples of exercises you can do without a gym membership or expensive equipment are push-ups, skipping rope, stretches, and crunches. In as little as 10 minutes a day, you'll notice a huge difference in how you look and feel.

Get plenty of rest. The amount of rest each person needs varies. The important thing is that you make it a priority to get to bed early enough that your body gets adequate rest. If you feel groggy every morning, consider going to bed earlier or finding a way to get in a short 15 to 30 minute power nap during the afternoon.

When you put these tips into practice, starting today, you'll experience a greater sense of vitality and self-confidence. With these simple techniques, the only thing that stands between you and the new fit you is action!

Helpful Affirmations for Losing Weight Fast

1. My weight loss goals are attainable.
2. My accomplishments include great triumphs in school, my career, and family matters.
3. Weight loss may be a challenge, but I know that my weight loss goal can be achieved just as I tackle other challenges in my life and win!
4. For a driven person like me, losing weight is more like a game rather than a burden. Each pound I lose is a sign of my strength and determination.
5. By placing such a positive spin on my efforts to lose weight, I increase both my confidence and my will to succeed.
6. My weight loss goals are perfectly achievable. I set a

reasonable timeline to lose weight and milestones to let me know how far I have come. Each time I reach a milestone, I treat myself to a movie or a gift unrelated to food.

7. Rewarding my achievements, no matter how small, gives me the motivation to keep on going.

8. I can have my cake and eat it too. But, I always make sure that it is angel food cake with a natural fruit topping! Choices like this let me enjoy the sweets I crave in healthier, smaller-calorie ways. The more I learn about food, the more pleasing choices I can find.

9. Like a game, I can find ways to prevent me from sabotaging myself, and win! Just as I can find tasty foods that are healthy, I also find fun ways to exercise.

10. With my positive mindset, the pounds just seem to be melting off! I am eating healthily, exercising regularly, and controlling my cravings.

11. Today, I keep my eye on the prize: fitting into my skinny jeans! I am actively working towards regaining the beach body that I once displayed proudly.

Self-Reflection Questions:

1. Am I losing weight to please myself or someone else?

2. Am I truly overweight or am I simply striving for perfection?

3. How can I curb cravings to stay strong in times of

weakness?

The Dream Dress Method

Every year, around the end of December, a lot of us are googling our asses off, hoping for some new breakthrough in the weight loss world,but every year, we pretty much discover the same thing: if we want to drop the pounds, we've got to move more and eat less.

Enter the "dream dress" method of weight loss, in which you purchase a beautiful dress or other outfit that you just LOVE and cannot wait to wear. The catch? You buy it in the size you WANT to be, not the size you are now.

No matter if you're currently sporting a 22 and looking to squeeze into a 2.

I'm sure you're not surprised that I have a small problem with this one, because I think that if you can't really love yourself as you are, right now, you'll never find real happiness anyway.

But inspiration can be good for weight loss. It can literally mean the difference between success and failure.

And there's nothing wrong with a little inspiration, obviously which is likely why so many fit pros are suggesting that we buy a "dream dress" or an outfit that is the ideal size for us.

The Dream Dress Method: How it can work in the real world for real women

Now, I can see how this could work. It HAS worked for me personally in the form of "dream jeans," actually.

But when it did work, it was literally when. I bought a pair of jeans that was only one or two (when I was sort of "between" sizes). That's because:

A. If you can't even get it over your big toe, it's going to feel like a goal you can't meet.
B. Fashion changes so quickly. If you're serious about wearing it this season, best to choose something that'll only take a few pounds to fit.
C. This allows you to go out and get another little bit of inspiration when you fit into the current one. It offers an instant reward that becomes motivation for the next weight loss goal.

So, how about you? Have you ever bought a "dream dress" and if so, did you ever manage to fit into it?

Easy Ways to Boost Your Metabolism

1. Thin and healthy people eat breakfast. You should too.

The morning meal jump starts your metabolism and helps to prevent binging later in the day. A cup of coffee does not count – the caffeine and added sugar may give you a bit of energy and suppress your appetite for a little while it is sure to backfire into severe hunger and you will be more likely to overeat later. Breakfast should include complex carbohydrates like whole grain (granola or oatmeal), along with some protein and fat (low-fat yogurt or milk), will keep your energy levels even and hunger in check.

2. Keep eating throughout the day.

Get into the habit of eating every three to four hours or at least four times a day. Eating frequently stabilizes blood sugar, when blood sugar drops too low you want to eat…a lot. By keeping your blood sugar stable you can control your appetite and keep you metabolic rate high. When you go many hours without eating your body will compensate by slowing down to conserve energy…this effect hurts your weight loss efforts.

3. No meat, no eat. That is, eat your protein. It can be meat or veggie-based–doesn't matter. Just eat it.

Protein will help to reduce your appetite, it takes more energy and time to digest, in effect you feel full longer than eating carbohydrates alone. Research shows that eating more protein can help you lose weight without cutting calories. Try these protein possibilities: turkey on whole wheat; hummus and pita; vegetarian chili; fruit and nuts; or protein snack bars that contain 12 or more grams of protein.

4. Listen to your body—only eat if you're truly hungry.

Many of us grab a snack for quick energy when we are feeling tired. But do not confuse true hunger with fatigue. If you are feeling tired go for a 15-20 minute brisk walk. This will raise your heart rate and give you a boost of energy. Follow it up with a large glass of cool water. If you are truly hungry have a protein and complex carbohydrate rich snack like; whole wheat crackers and peanut butter or cheese.

5. You've gotta eat ENOUGH to keep your body fueled up.

Eating too little slows your body's metabolism the same way eating too infrequently does. If you want to lose weight, do not slash your calories too drastically. Instead, cut out some of the extras in your diet – things like soda, juice, packaged goods or candy. Processed foods tend to be high in fat and calories and low in vitamins, minerals and fiber.

Fitness Mission: Move Your Body for 10 Minutes

"To keep the body in good health is a duty, otherwise we shall not be able to keep our mind strong and clear." ~ Buddha

In my experience, starting a workout program hard and fast

after months (or years) of couch surfing never works out well. So, if you haven't worked out in a while and today's your first day, the mission is simple: move your body for ten minutes. Some ideas:

- Walking
- Swimming
- Dancing/Belly Dancing
- Workout video
- Deep-clean a room
- Roller skate

If you've been working out for awhile, try adding ten minutes of activity to your day. Go for a walk around the block, dance like no one's watching or try the YouTube Workout Challenge.

Fitness Mission: YouTube Workout Challenge

I recently discovered the wonders of YouTube workout videos. There is a huge variety of videos out there, offering nearly every type of workout. So I thought, why not save money and try new things? That's why each day, I suggest you select one workout video from YouTube to get you started or to inspire you to try something new.

Just hit YouTube and type in "10 minute workout" or something similar and try it out.

How'd you do on today's mission? Share your experiences in the comments section, below. Don't forget to add your fitness notes to your Bliss Book.

Fitness Mission: Drink 8 Glasses of Water Today

One reason many people feel tired is that they're actually dehydrated.

Studies show that most people don't drink enough water throughout the day.

If you ask me, that could account for a lot of the exhaustion that leads to lack of activity and overeating.

(Plus, its a proven fact that when you don't drink enough water, your body actually retains water--it's sort of "afraid" to let go of what it's got for fear you won't replenish it. So, you appear more bloated.)

Next time you're tired, try drinking a glass of water, and try to stay hydrated throughout the day to maintain your energy levels.

"It's generally not a good idea to use thirst alone as a guide for when to drink," says a Mayo clinic expert. "By the time you become thirsty, you may already be slightly dehydrated."

Besides just being a healthier way to go, staying hydrated can actually aid in your weight loss efforts.

A 2010 study found that "obese dieters who drank two cups of water before each meal lost 5 pounds more than a group of dieters who didn't increase their water intake," according to Discovery News. "A year later, the water-drinkers had also kept more of the weight off."

So here's your mission:

Get your eight glasses in today!

Tips to Get It Done

1. Drink a glass of water before every cup of coffee or other beverage you drink.
2. Have one when you wake up in the morning, before anything else.
3. Have one before each meal (it'll help you feel full faster, too!).
4. Carry a water bottle with you and sip all day long.
5. Add lemon or decaf tea to your water if you can't drink it plain.

Do you drink eight glasses of water each day? If so, share your tips on how you get it done. If not, will you start today?

Fitness Mission: Get Your Sexy (Fitness) On!

I don't know about you, but I am totally loving this whole new "sexy fitness" craze that seems to be going on lately. From pole dancing classes to Flirty Girl Fitness and Carmen Electra's stripper fitness stuff, you almost can't get away from it.

See, we women are far more likely to succeed in getting and staying fit if we feel sexy--and these types of classes and videos are a big hit across the country for a reason.

Sexy fitness has even hit the Midwest. I was thrilled to find out that there is a new sexy fitness gym and cafe that just opened near me in January. This one was started by a pretty cool lady who has her whole vision and mission figured out--and I freaking LOVE IT! I can't wait to check it out.

From an article I wrote about my local studio, K.I.S.S. Fitness Cafe and Spa, for Florissant Patch:

K.I.S.S. stands for "Keep It Sexy Sistas," according to the company's website, and Smith said she was inspired by her mother's battle with obesity. In addition to starting her own workout program when she was just 15, Smith said that after seeing her mother lose her life due to weight-related health issues, she vowed to make a difference in the lives of others who struggle with obesity.

"Our approach to fitness is we make fitness fun," says the

company motto. "Lose the Excuses and Lose the Weight. If you are alive you can get stronger, healthier and sexier."

Did I mention that I LOVE it? Because I do. :) But let's get back on track, shall we?

Flirty-Girl Fitness Workout

Visit YouTube and search for the 10-minute Flirty Girl Fitness chair dance workout. It'll be fun! And who knows maybe it'll just spice up your sex life! :)

Fitness Mission: Flinging Off the Flabby Arm Fat

Since I've been losing weight, I've been feeling a lot better about the way my body looks and feels, but as my journey is a continuing one, I still have certain areas that I'm working on improving.

One of those is my upper arms. While I agree that they look/looked tremendously better than they once did, they are/were still a little plump and a little flabbier than I'd like.

So, for my personal challenge, I added a new goal: to tone up my flabby arms. And while we all know how important diet is when it comes to getting rid of flab, we should also remember how much shapelier (and healthier) it is to have a little lean muscle in there. I'm still working on it, and you can too!

Tone Up Flabby Arms With Exercise

Whether you're doing it to be healthier or you're doing it to be hotter (or both, like me), I invite you to join me in adding in a special daily workout (just a few minutes a day will do!) designed to tone up flabby arms.

Since I'm frugal (AKA cheap), I've collected a few free workout videos, each of which features exercises to tone up flabby arms over on YouTube. You can do the same.

Pick one (or more) and give it a shot!

Chapter 7: Final Notes for Your Own Project Blissful

How to Stay Motivated When You Have a LOT to Lose

When you've got a lot of weight to lose like I did, staying "on-plan" consistently can seem daunting.

I spent a lot of years trying to figure out how to stay motivated, and eventually, I got it. I lost 100 pounds (and counting—I've lost about 110 now and have a few more to go!).

But here's the good news. While my journey thus far has taken more than two years, I haven't spent a lot of that time feeling deprived, left out or unhappy.

I've changed the way I perceive myself and the world around me, and as a result, I've been able to take my time and learn to listen to my body.

Yet, even today, from time to time, I get on the scale regularly to make sure I'm moving in the right direction, as slow as the going is.

If I notice that the number goes up more than a pound or so (three during PMS week), I take notice and take action.

Over time, I've come up with a few weight loss motivation tips that really do work.

I stay motivated to continue my healthier lifestyle choices every day, one day at a time, thanks to my fail-safe plan that sort of developed naturally as I made the changes to both my lifestyle and my perception.

Sitting is the New Smoking

Can Exercise Make Up for a Whole Day of Sitting?

Many of us spend most of the day sitting down. You commute to work and likely sit in an office or cubicle during the day. Even if you drive a truck, you still spend a great deal of time sitting.

Find out why sitting for extended periods of time is bad for you:

> **Study #1.** A 2012 analysis of 18 different studies concluded that *those who sat for the longest periods of time were twice as likely to develop diseases such as diabetes and heart disease,* when compared to people who didn't sit as much.

> **Study #2.** An American Cancer Society study found that women who sit for more than 6 hours per day were

40% more likely to die during the course of the study than those who sat for less than 3 hours per day.

Men in the study were approximately 20% more likely to die under the same conditions.

Study #3. An inactivity researcher at the Pennington Biomedical Research Center did a study with rats that were forced to be inactive.

It was discovered that the leg muscles of inactive rats immediately lost over 75% of their ability to remove lipoproteins from the blood.

The same researcher conducted a study with 14 human volunteers who were young and physically fit. Within 24 hours of being sedentary, the volunteers had a 40% reduction in their insulin's ability to process glucose.

The Benefits of Exercise

No one is disputing the benefits of exercise. *There have been more than 40 studies in scientific literature documenting that the risk of cardiovascular disease can be cut by 30 to 50% when people partake in moderate exercise.* Some of the benefits of exercise include:

Weight loss

Increased overall health and a reduction in numerous

diseases and health issues

Elevated mood

Increased energy

Better sleep

Exercise Alone Isn't Enough to Undo the Damage Caused by Prolonged Sitting

Despite the benefits, exercise alone isn't enough to counteract the damage done by excessive sitting. So, what can be done if exercising isn't enough?

If you exercise regularly, continue to do so. If you're not exercising, start now. However, there

are some additional things you can do to prevent the damage done by prolonged sitting.

Implement these suggestions for getting up and moving more often:

> **Add variety to your day. *OSHA recommends mixing some non-computer-related tasks into your workday.*** Although you may need to spend some time sitting at the computer, find other tasks that require you to get up and walk around.

Consider using an exercise ball instead of a chair.
Because an exercise ball is unstable, it requires you to balance yourself using various stabilizer muscles in your legs and core.

Sitting on an exercise ball is good for your back and it helps keep your spine in proper alignment.

Get up and stand at your desk. If you have to be at your desk all day, there's no rule that prevents you from standing up. Activating your muscles gets the blood flowing.

Conventional wisdom would have us believe that getting a decent amount of exercise would offset the negative effects of prolonged sitting. However, exercise alone isn't the answer. So, make some adjustments today and lessen the amount of sitting you do. Your body will thank you.

Discover This Surprising New Ingredient for Exercise Motivation

Exercise motivation comes in many forms, from managing health conditions to wanting to look good for a high school reunion. Now, researchers have found an especially powerful resource by tapping into emotional memories.

A recent study found that asking people to remember previous workouts significantly increased the amount of exercise they did the next day. Happy memories had the strongest effect, but even unpleasant memories provided some inspiration.

Maybe you're struggling to stick with your aerobic classes or you just want an additional boost. Try these ideas for creating and using memories that will make you want to get moving.

Creating Memories for Exercise Motivation

- **Plan a vacation.** Play golf in Scotland or go scuba diving in the Caribbean. Bring home special memories that you'll love to revisit.
- **Take the scenic route.** *Make the most of your surroundings at home.* Jog along a wooded trail in your local park. Play volleyball at the beach. Buy a colorful yoga mat.
- **Engage all your senses.** Enjoy your workouts to the fullest. Buy a soft fluffy towel. Play your favorite tunes.
- **Make it social.** Everything becomes more unforgettable when you share it with others. Start a softball team at the office. Spend the weekend skiing with your family. *Find a workout buddy.* When someone else is counting on you, it's harder to make excuses when you've arranged to exercise.
- **Pay attention.** It's difficult to recall many details about

your time on the treadmill if your eyes are glued to a TV screen. Try activities that encourage more mindfulness, like Tai Chi.

- **Challenge yourself**. Striving to reach ambitious, but feasible, goals builds happiness and self- esteem. Work with a tennis coach or increase the mileage on your morning run.
- **Avoid injury.** At the same time, pleasant conditions provide the best motivation. Reduce your chances of getting burned out or sidelined by a sprained ankle or sore back. *Watch for signs of overtraining, and follow safety guidelines for any sport or exercise activity.*

Using Memories for Exercise Motivation

- **Keep a journal.** Putting things in writing makes past events more vivid. Record significant moments so you can read them later.
- **View pictures.** Images make a strong impression. Snap pictures with your phone or carry around a small digital camera so you can photograph yourself being active.
- **Learn to visualize.** Conjure up a mental image of fun times and outstanding achievements. Picture how you looked spinning around on the dance floor or scoring on the basketball court.
- **Break it down.** *If you've ever studied for a test or*

memorized a long password, you know the value of dividing information into smaller chunks. Trace your workouts from warm up to cool down.

- **Talk it over.** Solidify your memories by discussing them. Go out for coffee with your fitness buddy. It will give you both an opportunity to rehash your training sessions and benefit from each other's perspectives.
- **Make a morning resolution.** *You'll accomplish more by making frequent resolutions,* rather than waiting for New Year's. Start each day by forming an intention. Maybe you'll decide to swim laps during your lunch hour or sign up for tango classes.
- **Review at bedtime.** Monitor your progress to stay on track and sharpen your memories. Set aside time to evaluate what's working for you and what you want adjust.
- **Repeat and repeat.** Memories grow stronger with practice over extended time periods. *You're more*
- *likely to renew your gym membership if you give yourself regular reminders of all the benefits, such as controlling your weight and toning your muscles.*

Take a trip down memory lane the next time you're having trouble talking yourself into going to the gym. Memories can be one more tool for recharging your exercise motivation.

One Last Thing: My Long-Term, Fail-Safe, Stay-on-Plan

Weight Loss Motivation Tips

Forgive Yourself First

If you fall off-plan and find yourself backsliding into old, unhealthy habits, your first instinct might be to belittle yourself, beat yourself up, even to punish yourself.

One woman I know will literally starve herself for 24 hours for each "slip-up" she has on her plan to exercise and lose weight.

For example, at a birthday party, she indulged in a tiny piece of cake.

The next day, she worked out for 3 hours and refused to eat a thing.

The problem with this kind of behavior is twofold—besides being completely unhealthy and slowing down your metabolism, it's not a lifestyle that can be continued forever without serious consequences.

Rather than beat yourself up, just forgive yourself, love yourself that much more, and move forward on your plan.

Remind Yourself Why

You started this journey for a reason. Whether you wanted to live longer, be hotter, get healthier, play with your kids, have better sex, wear better clothes—or all of the above and more, make a list of reasons you're trying to get in shape.

Review the list anytime you feel yourself falling back into your old, unhealthy habits and really dig into the WHY of it all. Doing so can really renew your motivation in a big way.

Go Back to Basics

When I started this journey, I started small. I love me some baby steps! I made one change per week—first, I started tracking my food (not necessarily restricting, just becoming aware of what's really going into my mouth).

Once I got comfortable with that, a week or two later, I started keeping track of my water consumption and making sure I was getting in at least my eight glasses per day.

I kept making one small change at a time, and before I knew it, I'd lost 100 pounds!

So, if you find yourself slipping up, go back and remind yourself how you got started and get back to basics. For me, that's tracking my food again and drinking my water.

Look Back (at How Far You've Come Already)

One excellent way to remind yourself why you need to stay on track is to remind yourself how far you've already come, or of where you want to go.

You can do this with your own side-by-side before/during/after photos, or just look at old photos of your "old self."

It doesn't matter if your old self is sitting there reading this post and trying to find motivation, or if you've already lost a bunch of weight and are just trying to stay on track.

Anytime I see my own before/during photos, I am quickly reminded of why I need to continue on my path.

And before I had my own before and during photos, I used older pics of myself and photos of women I call "body idols"– otherwise known as women who were at my ideal weight and who also had a similar body structure and height.

One more tip - MyBodyGallery.com is a great place to find your own body idols, if you haven't already. (It's where I found some of mine!) Visual motivation can really open your eyes (pun intended) and keep you moving in the right direction.

About the Author

Angela Atkinson is a journalist who also happens to be a Certified Life Coach. Starting in 2011, Atkinson managed to lose more than 100 pounds and has kept it off for more than three years so far.

Along with her solution-focused life coaching experience, Atkinson's love of writing offers her the unique ability to share a new understanding of how life works for a whole new generation.

Atkinson's publishing resume is vast and varied and includes several years' experience in online journalism, including hard reporting as well as functioning as an editor in various iterations over the years.

In her life coaching practice, Atkinson's clients enjoy her personalized approach that allows and encourages them to become the best possible versions of themselves and to succeed in doing what they love most.

As you can see when you visit the freebies page at QueenBeeing.com, Atkinson's online daily magazine for women, she's all about paying it forward.

Other Books By Angela Atkinson

See the Most Current List at www.BooksAngieWrote.com

On Weight Loss and Self-Esteem

- Project Blissful: Your Whole Life Guide to Misery-Free Weight Loss That Really Works
- 227 Super-Simple, Super-Sexy Summer Slim-Down Strategies: The Smart Girl's Guide to a Very Sexy Summer (Project Blissful)

On Personal Success and Getting What You Want In Life

- 127 Powerfully Simple Life Hacks: Easy Ways to Empower Yourself and Improve Your Life in 30 Days or Less (Project Blissful)
- 69 INSTANT MANIFESTATION SECRETS: Quick and Easy Life Hacks for Remarkable Success (Project Blissful Book 4
- Here Are The Keys to Explosive Personal Power: How to Stop Being a Doormat and Instantly Start Living the Life You Deserve (Project Blissful Book 3)
- 127 Powerfully Simple Ways to Be Really, Really Happy: Proven Happiness Hacks for Busy People (Project Blissful Book 8)

On Career Success

- <u>163 Simply Powerful Career Hacks Anyone Can Use: Get Where You Want to Go In Your Career, One Easy Step at a Time (Project Blissful Book 5)</u>
- <u>The Practical Freelance Writer's Guide to Author Websites: How to Build, Manage and Promote a Freelance Writer Website (2010)</u>

On Narcissism and NPD

- <u>It's Not Supposed to Hurt: Overcoming Toxic Love and Narcissism in Relationships</u>
- <u>Your Love is My Drug: How to Shut Down a Narcissist, Detoxify Your Relationships & Live the Awesome Life You Really Deserve, Starting Right Now</u>
- <u>Take Back Your Life: 103 Highly-Effective Strategies to Snuff Out a Narcissist Gaslighting and Enjoy the Happy Life You Really Deserve (Detoxifying Your Life)</u>

On Love and Marriage Relationships

- <u>The Hot Wife Starter Kit: A Quick-Launch Guide to Getting Your Sexy Back, Starting Today (The Hot Wife Guides Book 1)</u>
- <u>How to Be a Hot Wife: Become the Kind of Wife Every Man Wants to Marry (And Every Woman Secretly Wants to Be): A Step-by-Step Guide to the Beautiful</u>

Life for Married Women (Hot Wife Guides Book 2)

Connect With Life Coach Angela Atkinson

Here are some ways we can connect:

- Email (angyatkinson@gmail.com)
- Twitter (@angieatkinson)
- Facebook (https://facebook.com/angelamatkinson)
- LinkedIn: https://www.linkedin.com/in/angieatkinson
- Google +: https://plus.google.com/+AngieAtkinson/posts
- Blog: QueenBeeing.com

www.ingramcontent.com/pod-product-compliance
Lightning Source LLC
Chambersburg PA
CBHW070400290526
45790CB00004B/1579